Head Injury: The Facts

My Articles* on Living with Brain Injury

By craig lock

*The most liked ones

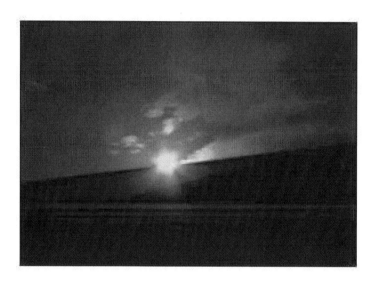

Dedication

A "labour of love" dedicated to all of you,
Marie, Sean and Gareth

You "guys and a gal" have made my 'little'
life a glorious happening"

c (November 2014)

Submitter's Note

Articles in this "little" book (booklet) sourced from my various Amazon books, *My Story, My 'Little' Life, Living with Head Injury, Who Wants to be Normal Anyway and An Open Book 3,* As well as my Wordpress blog at www.headbraininjury.wordpress.com and www.livingwithheadinjury.wordpress.com

All may be **freely reproduced**.

I hope you may find them helpful to you in better undersdanding what is often termed "the hidden handicap."

Craig

"We share what we know, so that we all may grow."

The various books* that Craig "felt inspired to write" are available at http://www.amazon.com/-/e/B005GGMAW4

http://www.amazon.com/s/ref=la_B005GGMAW4_sr?rh=i%3Abooks&field-author=Craig+Lock
https://www.createspace.com/pub/simplesitesearch.search.do?sitesearch_query=%22craig+lock%22&sitesearch_type=STORE

http://www.creativekiwis.com/index.php/books
and http://goo.gl/vTpjk

All proceeds go to needy and underprivileged children -

MINE!

CONTENTS

CONTENTS

*

Do not what you can't do – stop what you CAN do… best!

"I do not bewail what I have lost, because I am at peace with myself. I have fought a hard battle, given it my best, and won far more that I or anyone else ever thought I would. I ask only that other brain damaged people be given the chance to fight their battles too, and to find out for themselves what their unique potential is."
– Frederick Linge

From
www.livingwithheadinjury.wordpress.com/tag/frederick-r-linge/

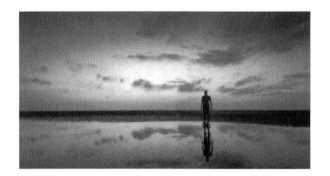

Craig has a close personal interest in this area and has been researching and studying in this field for nearly twenty years stemming from a long-standing and serious closed head injury. He hopes that by sharing that it will make some difference in those lives affected by brain injury.

Craig likes (no, rather loves) to share knowledge and insights from his life experiences to try and help others through simple encouragement. He hopes that by sharing this information, it will make some difference in those lives affected by brain injury.

Craig's new book *Living with Head Injury*: (from 'My Story') [Paperback] is available at http://www.amazon.com/Living-Head-Injury-My-Story/dp/1491063041/ (also available in Kindle format)

"We share what we know... so that we all may grow."

The various books* that Craig "felt inspired to write" (including those on head and brain injury, as well as his story) are available at http://www.amazon.com/-/e/B005GGMAW4

http://www.amazon.com/s/ref=la_B00 5GGMAW4_sr?rh=i%3Abooks&field-author=Craig+Lock https://www.createspace.com/pub/simplesitesear ch.search.do?sitesearch_query=%22craig+lock% 22&sitesearch_type=STORE

All proceeds go to needy and underprivileged children - MINE!

Don't worry about the world ending today... as it's already tomorrow in scenic and tranquil 'little' New Zealand

*

1.Head Injury: A Practical Guide: You are an Expert Already...

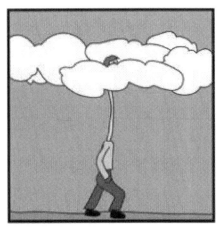

Article Title: Head Injury: A Practical Guide: You are an Expert Already...
Author: Trevor Powell
Submitted by: Craig Lock
Category (key words): Head injury, brain injury, neuro-psychology, Headway
Web site: http://www.headway.org.uk
Submitter's web sites: http://www.amazon.com/-/e/B005GGMAW4http://www.amazon.com/

LIVING-BRAIN-INJURY-STORY-ebook/dp/B005IQMC0W/
http://www.amazon.com/s/ref=la_B005GGMAW4_sr?rh=i%3Abooks&field-author=Craig+Lock&sort=relevance&ie=UTF8&qid and http://goo.gl/vTpjk

Other Articles by Craig are available at: http://www.selfgrowth.com/articles/user/15565 andhttp://www.ideamarketers.com/library/profile.cfm?writerid=981

(Personal growth, self help, writing, internet marketing, words of inspiration, "spiritual, spiritual writings" (how "airey-fairey"), and money management – how boring now, Craig!)

Publishing Guidelines:

I hope that the following piece may be informative to others (with acknowledgment to Trevor Powell and Headway, please (http://www.headway.org.uk). If it helps anyone "out there in the often very difficult, but always amazing 'journey of life' in any way, then we're very happy.

"We share what we know, so that we all may grow."

*

HEAD INJURY: YOU ARE AN EXPERT ALREADY...

Part of the text is reproduced by kind permission of Trevor Powell from his book *Head Injury: A Practical Gu*ide.

The cognitive effects of a brain injury affect the way a person thinks, learns and remembers. Different mental abilities are located in different parts of the brain, so a head injury can damage some, but not necessarily all, skills such as speed of thought, memory, understanding, concentration, solving problems and using language.

The cognitive system can be divided up into six separate areas:

Memory

Memory is not one thing or one skill on its own. It is easily damaged by brain injury because there are several structures within the brain which are involved in processing information, storing it and retrieving it. Damage to those parts of the brain on which these abilities depend can lead to poor memory. Problems with memory is a complex subject and is covered in more depth in a separate section.

Headway has produced a publication Memory Problems After Brain Injury that provides further information.

Attention and Concentration

A reduced concentration span is very common after head injury, as is a reduced ability to pay attention to more than one task at the same time. These problems are usually caused by damage to the frontal lobe. Attentional problems tend to get worse when the person is tired, stressed or worried. When there are problems with concentration, other skill areas can be affected. It is difficult to follow instructions, plan ahead, be organised and so on, when there is a problem concentrating. Working in a place with as few distractions as possible can help and, as concentration improves, distractions can be increased. In this way, someone can slowly learn to concentrate better in a world which is crowded with distracting sights and sounds.

Speed of Information Processing
Slowing down the speed at which the brain performs the task of information processing is often due to 'diffuse axonal damage' caused by a shake up of all of the pathways the brain uses to transmit messages. This results in problems such as not understanding fast speech, being unable to absorb instructions first time around, and not being able to quickly formulate a reply to a question. To improve the speed of information processing, it is advisable to keep mentally stimulated at the right level to avoid overload.
Executive Functions – Planning, Organising, Problem Solving
Damage to the frontal lobe can affect these skills, resulting in a subtle set of deficits which have been called 'Dysexecutive Syndrome'. This covers problems in making long-term plans, goal setting and initiating steps to achieve objectives. The ability to stand back and take an objective view of a situation may be lacking, as may the

ability to see anything from another person's point of view. If the person is aware that this is a problem, then encouragement and direct feedback can be given to help the person modify their behaviour. It is useful to try to create structure in otherwise unstructured situations, by breaking down any task into specific tasks, perhaps using checklists. Flexible thinking is made up of both divergent thinking (thinking outwards or generating ideas from a single point) and convergent thinking (thinking inwards, taking ideas and summarising them). Exercises which practice these skills not only improve ability but help to identify difficulties and improve awareness.

Visuo-Spatial and Perceptual Difficulties

Organs such as ears and eyes may be working perfectly well, but the part of the brain which makes sense of incoming information from these sources may not be working properly. This gives rise to several different types of difficulty. Problems in judging distances, spatial relationships and orientation can mean, for example, that a person may bump into furniture that they have seen, but have misjudged where it is in relation to themselves. Sometimes a person will have a problem where one side of whatever they are looking at is not seen (visual neglect). A person may only eat half the food on their plate, or read only halfway the across the page. The ability to recognise something viewed from a different or unusual angle can be lost. This can also apply to sounds as well as vision. Building objects or drawing them from component parts such as coloured block may be very hard.

Language Skills

Problems with language loss can be either receptive such that no sense can be made of what is heard or read, or expressive which means it is not easy to find the right words to say or write. Difficulties with these areas are known as aphasia. When both problems are present the condition is known as 'global aphasia'. There is a special area on the left side of the brain concerned with producing speech (Broca's area which is located between the frontal and temporal lobes) and another area for understanding the speech of others (Wernickes's area which is located further back between the temporal and parietal lobes). These two are connected by numerous pathways but are quite distinct. It is useful to remember that the brain skills which produce and understand speech are different to the ability to make the sounds of language. The latter can be due to problems with the muscles in the throat and mouth, and more detailed information is given in the section on physical effects after head injury.

A publication titled Communication Problems after Brain Injury is available which describes the common problems and gives hints and tips on dealing with them.

Other organisations can help, such as Speakability.

EMOTIONAL EFFECTS:

Everyone who has had a head injury can be left with some changes in emotional reaction and behaviour. These are more difficult to see than the more obvious problems such as those which affect movement (a physical effect) and speech (a cognitive effect), for example, but can be the most difficult for the individual concerned and their family to deal with.

Headway has produced publications to help and advise on many of the problems outlined below. There are more than twenty titles covering subjects such as Psychological Effects of Brain Injury and Personal and Sexual Relationships Following Brain Injury

Headway's network of local Groups and Branches are an excellent source of advice and support for the head injured person and members of the family by people who have experienced these difficulties at first hand, and can advise on coping strategies and treatment methods.

This subject is very large, and not everybody will experience all of the problems below. The severity of the problems will also vary.

Agitation

Explosive Anger and Irritability

For example, exaggerated angry reaction to apparently minor annoyances.

Direct damage to the frontal lobes, which is the part of the brain which controls emotional behaviour and tolerance of frustration, can create emotional lability. This means emotions can swing to extremes. The stress of coping with even minor crises, such as misplaced shoes or a noisy vacuum cleaner, can be too much and trigger an angry outburst. If these stresses can be identified, they may be able to be reduced.

Lack of Awareness and Insight

The mental ability to monitor personal behaviour and adjust it accordingly is a sophisticated skill contained in the frontal lobes of the brain. Damage to this area affects the ability to be self-aware, have insight into the effects of personal actions, show sensitivity or feel empathy. It also means that a person may not fully appreciate or understand the effect that the accident is having on their life, health or family. Involvement in a head injury support group can be very useful for meeting people at various stages of recovery, who can help a person recognise difficulties they may also be experiencing.

Impulsivity and Dis-inhibition

For example, speaking your mind no matter what the circumstances, touching people inappropriately, and not considering the consequences of any action.

This is the lack of ability to control either actions or speech, and is due to neurological damage to the frontal lobes. This problem often goes hand in hand with lack of awareness, and the person may not be aware of breaching any social rules or etiquette. A behavioural management system devised with the help of a neuro-psychologist can help improve the situation, and prevent a person developing unacceptable behaviour through habit.

Emotional Liability

This describes a person's tendency to laugh and cry very easily and to move from one emotional state to another very quickly.

Loss of control over emotions means the person has lost the ability to discriminate about when and how to express their feelings. This can be very tiring and embarrassing for family members to deal with, but in time a person can begin to re-learn emotional control.

Self-Centredness

For example, not showing any interest in family matters, and only being concerned with personal needs.

This can be partly due to direct brain injury affecting a person's ability to judge how another person is feeling, and may be partly due to a person becoming accustomed to the huge amount of attention focused on a head injury survivor while they were in hospital. The result can be very hard to cope with. It needs to be handled firmly to avoid a family feeling their effort and love are not appreciated.

Apathy and Poor Motivation

For example, no interest in hobbies enjoyed previously, or not being bothered to get out of a chair all day.

Lack of motivation or spontaneity, or apathy, is a direct result of brain injury to frontal lobe structures that concern emotion, motivation or

forward planning. Over time, lack
of motivation can lead to social isolation and lack
of pleasure. To help, activities can be broken
down into small steps to avoid overwhelming the
person.

Depression

For example, feeling there is no point in having
survived the accident, or thinking that everything
has changed for the worse.

Depression is a very common emotional reaction
which comes on in the later stages of
rehabilitation, often when a person realises the
full extent of the problems caused by the
accident. This can be seen as a good sign, that a
person is aware of the reality of the situation, and
is coming to term with the emotional
consequences. 'Healthy' depression can be
worked through in time, as adjustments are made.
If a person feels emotionally blocked and unable
to move on, professional counselling from
someone who understands head injury may be
helpful.

Anxiety

For example, panic attacks, nightmares, and
feelings of insecurity.

It is natural for people involved in a traumatic
experience to feel anxious afterwards. Loss of
confidence when faced with situations and tasks
which are difficult to cope with is also a pretty
normal reaction. However, long standing
problems can occur if difficult situations are
continually avoided, or if carers encourage

dependence rather than independence. Talking about fears and worries is very helpful, and adopting methods of staying calm under stress can reduce the effect of anxiety on everyday life.

Inflexibility and Obsessionality

For example, unreasonable stubbornness, obsessive pattern of behaviour such as washing or checking things, or fear of possessions being stolen.

The ability to reason must not be taken for granted. The roots of this type of rigid behaviour are in cognitive difficulties resulting from damage to the frontal lobes. The person can lose the ability to jump from one idea to another, and becomes 'stuck' on one particular thought. This type of behaviour is often made worse by anxiety or insecurity, so reassurance is helpful, as is trying to redirect attention to more constructive ideas and behaviour. This type of behaviour can be very irritating to family and friends, and often leads to social isolation.

Part of the text is reproduced by kind permission of Trevor Powell from his book Head Injury: A Practical Guide

Trevor Powell

*

"The task ahead of you can always be overcome by the power within you…and the seemingly

difficult path ahead of you is never as steep with
the great spirit that lies within you."
"When the world is filled with love, people's
hearts are overflowing with hope."
– craig
"Success to others may be apparent in what you
DO; but
significance, meaning and purpose lies, then
reveals itself
in what you ARE and BECOME down the 'river
of life' – how
and the spirit with which you face, then
overcome the daily
obstacles, the frequent trials and tribulations
along the
often rocky path-way of life's magical and
mysterious
journey.
Light your path brightly."
http://www.craiglockbooks.com
About the Submitter:
Craig has a close personal interest in this area
and has been researching and studying in this
field for nearly twenty years stemming from a
long-standing head injury. He hopes that by
sharing that it will make some difference in those
lives affected by brain injury. Craig likes to share
knowledge and insights from his life experiences
to try and help others through simple
encouragement. He hopes that by sharing this
information, it will make some difference in
those lives affected by head injury.

The various books that Craig "felt inspired to write" (including his books on head injury and 'My Story' are available at http://www.amazon.com/-/e/B005GGMAW4 http://www.amazon.com/LIVING-BRAIN-INJURY-STORY-ebook/dp/B005IQMC0W/ http://www.amazon.com/s/ref=la_B005GGMAW4_sr?rh=i%3Abooks&field-author=Craig+Lock&sort=relevance&ie=UTF8&qid and http://goo.gl/vTpjk

My book 'LIVING WITH HEAD/BRAIN INJURY (from 'MY STORY') is available at http://www.amazon.com/LIVING-BRAIN-INJURY-STORY-ebook/dp/B005IQMC0W/

The submitter's blogs (with extracts from his various writings: articles, books and new manuscripts) are at http://craigsblogs.wordpress.

"Together, one mind, one life at a time, let's see how many people we can impact, encourage, empower, uplift and perhaps even inspire to reach their fullest potentials."

This article may be freely reproduced electronically or in print. If through sharing a little of my experiences, it helps anyone "out there in the often very difficult, but always amazing 'journey of life' in any way, then I'm very happy.

PPS: Do not what you can't do – stop what you CAN do best!

2.Article Title: Some Cognitive Effects of Head Injury

Author: Craig Lock

Category (key words): head injury, brain injury, brain damage, neuro-psychology, medical information, medical resources

Web sites: http://www.amazon.com/-/e/B005GGMAW4http://www.creativekiwis.com/amazon.html andhttp://www.smashwords.com/profile/view/craiglock

The submitter's blogs (with extracts from his various writings: articles, books and new manuscripts) are
at www.headbraininjury.wordpress.com and http://craigsblogs.wordpress.com

Other Articles are available
at: http://www.selfgrowth.com/articles.html
(Personal growth, self help, writing, internet marketing, spiritual, 'spiritual writings' (how 'airey-fairey'), words of inspiration and money management, how boring now, craig!)

Publishing Guidelines: I hope that the following piece may be informative to others. This article may be freely reproduced electronically or in print. Although very personal, if through sharing a little of my experiences, it helps anyone "out there in the often very difficult, but always amazing 'journey of life' in any way, then I'm very happy.

We share what we know, so that we all may grow."

*

2.

SOME COGNITIVE EFFECTS OF HEAD INJURY:

by Craig Lock

"Compare it (your head) to a jelly in a bowl. The bowl is the skull – a strong, protective container – and the jelly (the brain) is nestled within. The skull is able to withstand many types of blows; but the brain is vulnerable to sudden swirling or rotating movements. Shake the bowl and see what happens to the jelly."

– Dr Don Mackie, Emergency Specialist(in New Zealand)

This extract (in note form) is from a chapter from my manuscript titled *MY STORY, MY DREAM available* at http://www.amazon.com/Ill-Do-It-My-Way/ *and as an e-book at* http://www.amazon.com/Ill-Do-It-Way-ebook/dp/B005GS6ZVO

Also LIVING WITH HEAD (BRAIN) INJURY (from 'MY STORY') * [Kindle Edition http://www.amazon.com/LIVING-BRAIN-INJURY-STORY-ebook/dp/B005IQMC0W/

#

Firstly ...extreme FATIGUE

* Wake up every morning feeling heavy-headed (very).

* fatigue – take frequent breaks and do the most demanding tasks first...even get exhausted reading a newspaper! So break the task into "bytes"...doing most of my reading "first thing" when I awaken early)

* in SA found telling stories very difficult – kept facts to a minimum. Write way better than I talk.

* muddled – making tea AND coffee for guests. Sugar, one two, milk??? Total confusion making for more than just myself. Ha ha (just ask my friends if it's true – a clue – they make the drinks)! So I put one thing away at a time, then finish. Single-minded FOCUS.

Not observant.

Visio-spatial organisation

short-term and visual memory (visual overload)

I have the ideal job (at long last!). Very part-time and flexible, work in my own time, take breaks when fatigued. Info overload (and change) is a real problem, when other things are going on – groups (avoid that!), etc.

WITH determination, self discipline one can achieve wonders.

*

THE EFFECTS OF FATIGUE:

I wake up every morning feeling exhausted, as if I haven't had a good night's rest. ALWAYS. A bit light-headed too – no very HEAVY-headed. It's hard to describe the feeling. I feel I could sleep for days, but force my self out of bed to do my daily tasks. However, the first 2-3 hours of the day are by far my best times for alertness and getting the most important tasks done (like sending out articles on the internet). Also get more tired as the day progresses. I need more rest and have to work my day around my "funny job(s)" – by taking frequent rests and walks. It's not at all <u>depression</u>, just REAL FATIGUE – a "heavy headed" feeling, a bit like

the "hung-over" feeling (not that I've had one for "moons" – thank goodness I don't drink much... what I be like then... a total zombie!).

* Wake up every morning feeling heavy-headed (very).

* fatigue – take frequent breaks and do the most demanding tasks first...even get exhausted reading a newspaper! So break the task into "bytes"...doing most of my reading "first thing" when I awaken early)(Repeated for effect, not light-headedness!)

On reflection, my Lifegrow <u>insurance</u> job in Cape Town, South Africa was perfect for me... It was liason/marketing/PR. Worked few hours early am, then socialised just 'cruisin around'. Only then I didn't know then what I now know....and how well it suited me. Thank goodness for the great people, who helped me to "success" (Nicola, Rethe, Tony and Ronnie). Then after "emigrating" everything, our entire worlds, came crashing down in Perth, Australia ...and the real struggles began. Yet God can do the most amazing things, work <u>miracles</u>... by turning our deeeepest scars in to the most brilliant stars.

Now many many years later after that trauma my current position selling subscriptions for Sky TV (very part-time) here in a small provincial NZ city suits me perfectly. Flexible hours working when I want out of the "corporate rat race" and doing it "totally my way" (even with the occasional 'Frank Spencer episode'!) . I've been doing it very successfully for over three and a half years (five now, now over ten!). It's my longest and best job in my entire "career" and I'm very happy here "*Dropped out in Godzone*" (the title of my second book, btw).
BE HAPPY too

craig Nov 2012
PS:
If you are interested, there's a great detailed

article by Dr Frederick Linge
at http://www.selfgrowth.com/articles/What Does it Feel Like to be Brain Damaged.html

It's also on this blog
at www.headbraininjury.wordpress.com
"Success to others may be apparent in what you DO; but
significance, meaning and purpose lies, then reveals itself
in what you ARE and BECOME down the 'river of life' – how
and the spirit with which you face, then overcome the daily
obstacles, the frequent trials and tribulations along the
often rocky path-way of life's magical and mysterious
journey.
Light **your** path brightly."'

"The task ahead of you can always be overcome by the power behind you...and the seemingly difficult path ahead of you is never as steep with the great spirit that lies within you."

*"When the world is filled with love, people's hearts are overflowing with **hope**."*
- craig

About the submitter:

Craig has a long-standing head injury and has been researching and studying in this field for nearly twenty years. He hopes that by sharing this information, it will make some difference in those lives affected by brain injury www.craiglockbooks.com www.selfgrowth.com/experts/craig_lock.html

The various books that Craig "felt inspired to write" are available at:http://www.amazon.com/-/e/B005GGMAW4 and http://www.creativekiwis.com/amazon.html

MY STORY, MY DREAM is available at http://www.amazon.com/Ill-Do-It-My-Way/and as an e-book at http://www.amazon.com/Ill-Do-It-Way-ebook/dp/B005GS6ZVO
Also LIVING WITH HEAD (BRAIN) INJURY (from 'MY STORY') * [Kindle Edition*http://www.amazon.com/LIVING-BRAIN-INJURY-STORY-ebook/dp/B005IQMC0W/*
The submitter's blogs (with extracts from his various writings: articles, books and new manuscripts) are at www.headbraininjury.wordpress.com and http://craigsblogs.wordpress.com

This article may be freely reproduced electronically or in print. If it helps anyone "out there in the often very difficult, but always amazing 'journey of life' in any way, then I'm very happy.

PPS

"Let's not what we can't do stop us from doing what we CAN do...best!"

3.Living with Long-Term Brain (Head) Injury

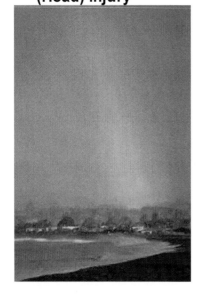

Article Title: Living with Long-Term Brain (Head) Injury
Submitted by: Craig Lock
Category (key words): Head injury, brain injury, William Fairbank, effects of brain/head injury, neuro-psychology, brain,

cognitive difficulties, medical information,
medical resources (enough there now, craig)
Web sites: www.williamfairbank.com
http://headbraininjury.wordpress.com/2014/08/03
/an-open-book-3-my-story/
http://www.amazon.com/Living-Head-
Injury-My-Story/dp/1491063041/
 http://www.amazon.com/-
/e/B005GGMAW4 andhttp://headbraininju
ry.wordpress.com/
The submitter's blogs (with extracts from his
various writings: articles, books and new
manuscripts) are
at https://livingwithheadinjury.wordpress.c
om/ andhttp://craigsblogs.wordpress.
Other Articles by Craig are available
at: http://www.selfgrowth.com/articles/user
/15565and http://www.ideamarketers.com/l
ibrary/profile.cfm?writerid=981
(Personal growth, self help, writing, internet
marketing, spiritual, 'spiritual writings' (how
'airey-fairey'), words of inspiration and
money management, how boring now,
craig!)

Publishing Guidelines:
I hope that the following piece may be
informative to others. This article may be
freely reproduced electronically or in print.
If it helps anyone "out there in the often very
difficult, but always amazing 'journey of life'
in any way, then we're very happy.

"We share what we know, so that we all may grow."

#

LIVING WITH LONG TERM BRAIN (HEAD) INJURY

INTRODUCTION

Here is some "info", that I summarised from a radio interview with a UK film-maker by the name of William Fairbank (http://www.williamfairbank.com) talking about the "hidden handicap, the silent epidemic". ("It could have been me speaking" . . . but not nearly as eloquently* as William!)

*big word, eh!

Head injury has become a common problem throughout the world. Many of the more severe injuries are related to road traffic and horse riding accidents. As an example, in Great Britain about 15 patients every hour are admitted to hospital for observation, because of head injury and every 2 hours one of these will die. Head injury is implicated in 1 of all deaths and 50% OF ROAD TRAFFIC ACCIDENT DEATHS. Head injury is particularly prevalent in the age group between 10 and 25. CONCUSSION has occurred, whenever patients cannot remember the actual blow that made them unconscious.

*

WILLIAM FAIRBANKS Interview with
Kathryn Ryan on National Radio (4th Feb
2010)

LONG-TERM BRAIN INJURY
"There is excellent medical care immediately
post-trauma. However, there is little follow-
up after the initial trauma. Every day I have
to come to terms with my brain injury, to
learn. I don't handle interruptions. It's like
being in a movie. Each person with a brain
injury is different...and is affected in
different ways. I do one thing at a time –
break into little tasks. I really live in the
present. No-one ever explained to me how to
cope, how to deal with everyday living. I had
to learn strategies for myself.
Difficulties in 'making connections':
I can only handle "one-on-one" situations. I
can't hold two thoughts in my mind at the
same time. A ringing phone will interrupt my
thought and sequence. I easily lose the 'flow'
of the task I was engaged in. Then I have
difficulty wondering what to do next! I have
to clear clutter to simplify my life. Get easily
'thrown' Head injured people are often self
absorbed. (Probably helps them cope with
life through focussing??)
NB Everyone with a head injury is affected
differently.

No-one can understand my problems, because I appear to be a lucid, intelligent man. I'm fine here now doing ONE thing. I want to contact artists: musicians, sculptors, poets, writers who have had a brain injury. So many people who have suffered a head injury write and draw; they channel it into some form of art.

Doctors don't understand brain injury and especially the effects, the cognitive difficulties people have; because the effects are so subtle (yet can have a huge effect on their lives). Head injury acts as a filter, a "block". It's such a fine-line brain-injured people have compared with normal-thinking people.

I can't visualise and have big problems with my short-term memory. It can be so FRUSTRATING (GRRRR) and often leads to mood swings and severe emotional problems.

Finally...
"Still **don't let what you can't do, interfere with what you CAN do (best)."**

"The important thing in life is not to triumph but to compete...it's not victory but combat...not to have vanquished but to have fought well...not winning but taking part."
— Pierre de Coubertin (French Educator,

primarily responsible for the revival of the
Olympic Games in 1894. 1863-1937)

Don't see head injury as a 'handicap', but
just another challenge to live with, work
around and overcome in the amazing
journey of life.

With knowledge comes understanding and
acceptance.

Shared by "information distributer and
incorrigible encourager" craig
"Success to others may be apparent in what
you DO; but significance, meaning and
purpose lies, then reveals itself in what you
ARE and BECOME down the 'river of life' –
how and the spirit with which you face, then
overcome the daily obstacles, the frequent
trials and tribulations along the often rocky
path-way of life's magical and mysterious
journey. Light your path brightly."
- craig

"The important thing in life is not to triumph
but to compete…it's not victory but
combat…not to have vanquished but to have
fought well…not winning but taking part."
— Pierre de Coubertin (French Educator,
primarily responsible for the revival of the
Olympic Games in 1894. 1863-1937)

PS: To end off, enjoy these thoughts...

*"We have it within; but we get it all from
without. There is a well-spring of
strength, wisdom, courage and
great imagination within each one of us;
but once we draw on this truth, it gets
watered from without, by a Higher Source
– the Source of Life and Love, which is God,
the very Ground of our Being."*

*When you can see no light at the end of the
tunnel, light your own candle and let your
light illuminate the world, like the radiance
from a window at midnight."
That's a metaphor, BTW"*

*"The task ahead of you can always be
overcome by the power within you...and the
seemingly difficult path ahead of you is
never as steep with the great spirit that lies
within you."*

*"When the world is filled with love, people's
hearts are overflowing with hope."*
– craig

About the Submitter:
Craig has a close personal interest in this
area and has been researching and studying
in this field for nearly twenty years

stemming from a long-standing head injury. He hopes that by sharing that it will make some difference in those lives affected by brain injury. Craig likes to share knowledge and insights from his life experiences to try and help others through simple encouragement. He hopes that by sharing this information, it will make some difference in those lives affected by brain injury.

Craig's new book *Living with Head Injury*: (from 'My Story') [Paperback] is available at http://www.amazon.com/Living-Head-Injury-My-Story/dp/1491063041/ (also available in Kindle format)

Also http://headbraininjury.wordpress.com/2014/08/03/an-open-book-3-my-story/

The various books that Craig "felt inspired to write" (including his books on head injury and 'My Story' are available at http://www.amazon.com/-/e/B005GGMAW4 http://www.smashwords.com/profile/view/craiglockwww.creativekiwis.com/in...www.lulu.com/craiglockand www.craigsbooks.wordpress.com

The submitter's blogs (with extracts from his various writings: articles, books and new manuscripts) are at https://livingwithheadinjury.wordpress.com/ andhttp://craigsblogs.wordpress.

"Together, one mind, one life at a time, let's see how many people we can impact, encourage, empower, uplift and perhaps even inspire to reach their fullest potentials."
This article may be freely reproduced electronically or in print. If through sharing a little of my experiences, it helps anyone "out there in the often very difficult, but always amazing 'journey of life' in any way, then I'm very happy.

1.What Does it Feel Like to be Brain Damaged?

Posted on September 18, 2013by craiglock

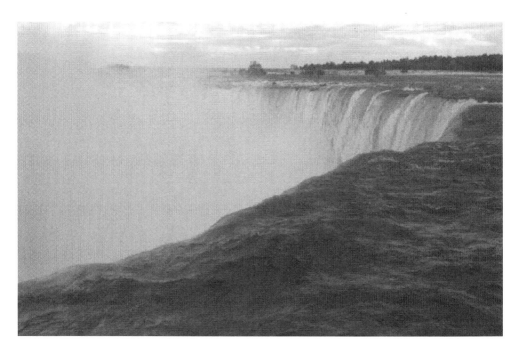

Article Title: What Does it Feel Like to be
Brain Damaged?
Author: Frederick R. Linge, Clinical
Psychologist
Submitted by: Craig Lock
Category (key words): head injury, brain
injury, neuro-psychology, brain
enhancement
Submitter's web
sites: http://www.amazon.com/-
/e/B005GGMAW4 andhttp://www.creativek
iwis.com/amazon.html
The submitter's blogs (with extracts from his
various writings: articles, books and new
manuscripts) are
at www.headbraininjury.wordpress.com and
http://craigsblogs.wordpress.com

Other Articles are available
at: http://www.selfgrowth.com/articles.html
Publishing Guidelines:
I hope that the following piece by Dr
Frederick Linge (with minor punctuation
and editing) may be informative and helpful
to others. This article may be freely
reproduced electronically or in print (with
acknowledgement to Dr Linge, please). If it
helps anyone "out there in the often very
difficult, but always amazing 'journey of life'
in any way (as it did myself and my wife in a
very difficult period of our life all those years
ago in Perth, Australia), then we're very
happy.

*"We share what we know, so that we all
may grow.*
*

What Does it Feel Like to be Brain Damaged?

By Frederick R. Linge, Clinical Psychologist

Introduction

It is generally accepted that people working
with individuals who have any type of
handicap, should have a certain amount of
empathy with their clients and should strive
to understand how their clients feel and
think. People working with those who are
brain damaged have a particularly hard time

doing so. One can have some understanding of what it means to be blind by simply closing one?s eyes; yet how can a normal person understand what it feels like to be brain damaged?

I am in the unusual position of being a trained clinical psychologist who suffered brain damage and who has slowly recovered most of my facilities. In other words, I have been on the outside looking in, and also, on the inside looking out at the world of the brain damaged person. At this point in my recovery, I have a foot in both worlds, for I can remember what it felt like to be completely normal intellectually, and also what it felt like when loss of function was at its worst.

Perhaps this informal and very subjective narrative may be of some help in assisting normal people to empathize a little better with the brain damaged individual. For, unfortunately, most brain damaged people are unable to explain precisely how they feel; those who have been brain damaged since birth, of course, have never had the experience of functioning normally and thus have no standard of comparison of their present state with that of others.

At the age of thirty-nine, I was an exceptionally healthy male with a keen interest in outdoor sports such as skiing, canoeing, and swimming. I had been a clinical psychologist for sixteen years and was married to a social worker; we had three children. I was active intellectually, reading a great deal both in and outside my field, and enjoyed classical music and playing the piano.

The Trauma

I have no memory of the head-on automobile collision that took place one spring evening. I have driven the same stretch of road innumerable times since then, listened to the testimony of witnesses, even examined official photographs of the wrecked vehicles; but nothing triggers any memory of the emotional responses. Hospital records indicate that I was admitted in critical condition, with a broken neck, fractured skull, broken jaw, broken ribs, multiple fractures of the right arm, splintered left leg and ankle, broken hip, internal injuries, numerous abrasions and contusions. The brain damage, which could be only partially assessed at first, was severe enough to render me totally unconscious for almost a week. I was paralyzed on the right side, and showed no response to visual, auditory or other stimuli. Heroic surgical procedures and the use of life support machinery kept me alive the first few days; but I was given little or no chance of surviving and it was thought that if I did survive, I might well do so as a human vegetable.

I have no memory of the first few weeks in the hospital's Intensive Care Unit. My wife was with me almost around the clock for the first two weeks and for several hours per day thereafter until I was discharged. She tells me that, even when seemingly unconscious, my body was constantly in motion, tugging at the traction, trying to move limbs immobilized by casts, testing out my limits of movement. On some level, it would seem that my body was fighting on its own, even when my brain was unable to function.

Early Communication Attempts

As the profound coma lifted at the end of the first week, my first response was to recognize, by smiling at familiar figures such as my wife, the children, and other relatives. At this time, my wife thinks I had regressed emotionally to almost an infantile state, wanting to touch her and the nurses, wanting to hold onto her hand and becoming agitated when she had to let it go, even for a moment.

At the same time, I showed a great deal of agitation and rage. Frequently, I would fight desperately to be free of the traction and would hit out angrily at those around me. When somehow or other, I managed to roll completely out of bed and land on the floor, cast, traction, broken neck and all, I was placed in a straight jacket and wrist restraints, and these added greatly to my emotional distress.

My family recalls that I seemed quite desperate to communicate and my failure to do so infuriated me as much as the physical immobility. I would try to write, but the script was almost illegible. Many letters were reversed, syllables were repeated over and over, and the meaning was garbled and incomprehensible. I am told that I would become so frustrated at people's inability to understand me, that I would stab the pencil through the paper, crumple it up, or hit out at those around me. Speech was, of course, out of the question, since I had a tracheotomy and was also on a respirator. I can only guess at the fear and confusion that must have filled me during those long, pain-filled weeks, during which I was unable to move, and unable to communicate in any way. Perhaps it is as well that I have no memory of them.

It was with the removal of the tracheotomy tubes and the restoration of my speech, that my confusion and agitation began slowly to subside. I have some hazy memories of this time. My first memory is that of the plastic surgeon removing wires from my jaws that had held them in place while the fractures healed. The intense pain seemed to jolt me into some contact with reality. I remember seeing the doctor as a gigantic, looming figure, although in reality he is a slight person.

Time and Reality Orientation

During this period, I had no awareness of time. I existed in a world of here and now. I was not even aware that such concepts of time existed. I knew who I was; but did not think of myself as being a child, a boy, or a man. My wife and my mother (who had died some years previously were both present in my thoughts and were indistinguishable to me. The staff of the hospital were also interchangeable shadowy figures. I remember feeling passive, accepting, acquiescent. People came and went, did things to me: I did not question them. I am told by my wife that during this period I was less physically agitated: calm, often dreamy, and seemed happy in a childlike sort of way, smiling frequently and making few demands.

On the day that I regained some consciousness, my wife constructed a large homemade calendar, which she placed beside my bed in clear view. On each visit, she would make a point of drawing my attention to the day of the week, the date of the month and the year, as well as the time displayed on the large wall clock near my bed. This seemed to have no effect at first. I would repeat the information after her, but forgot it immediately. It had no meaning for me.

One day, however, my mental clock began ticking again and the concept of time began to become significant. Somehow, I assimilated the fact that eight o'clock meant the end of visiting hours and my wife's departure, something I hated to have happen. One morning, I remember becoming quite agitated as the clock drew towards eight. Why isn't my wife here? It's almost eight and visiting hours are ending. When she laughed at me and informed me that it was eight in the morning, I remembered feeling foolish and embarrassed, and covering up as best I could: Oh yes, of course you're right. From that time onwards, I began to orient myself in time, frequently becoming confused, but making steady progress. It was in the area of daily time that I first began to realize that I had a deficit within myself, since those around me were clear-headed and confident about facts and I was not.

As the sequence of night and day became cleared, the large chronological picture began to come into focus, though with difficulty. Looking back, I know that, while I was in the early stages of recovery, I lost about ten years of memories. At first this did not matter to me... since past, present and future were all combined into a seamless here, now.

Nor was there a boundary between reality and fantasy. I cannot myself remember, but I am told that during the first weeks I was delusional and hallucinatory at times. A nurse's gown hanging behind the door became an intruder, ready to attack. Some delusions obviously served as an escape mechanism from the ever-present pain and physical restriction or served to explain to me why I was in the position that I was in. For example, I am told that I thought for some days that I was on an ocean liner with my wife bound on a pleasure cruise. Observation windows in the intensive care unit became portholes, nurses became stewardesses and so on, and my cubicle was a stateroom. Or, I would imagine I was on a desert island, surrounded by lapping waves.

Gradually, as I became more oriented and more aware that something had happened to me, the split between reality as seen by those around me and as I interpreted it, became more painful. I would argue with those around me in defence of my fantasies. Gradually, most of these died away; but the fantasy persisted that I was in the Kamloops hospital, where I had spent some months as a teenager...and that my parents were still alive and living in the family home near Kamloops, where I had grown up. I see now that this was my way of coping with the ten-year gap in my memory, a gap that I simply could not admit to myself at that point in my recovery.

The first breakthrough towards acceptance of reality came in a particularly poignant form. I had been asking with increasing vehemence for some days why my mother had not been to visit me and harassed my wife with demands that she do something about it. Too tender hearted to confront me with the fact that my mother was long dead, my wife tried to fob me off with various excuses. Quite suddenly, one day, I looked up at her and said in surprise and grief: 'What are we arguing about? My mother can't come to see me. She's dead.' I began to weep. Traumatic though this reliving of the grief of her <u>death</u> was, it was the beginning of a new stage of progress. From that moment on, I knew roughly where I stood in the stream of time. I had some grasp of the continuim of life and <u>death</u>, youth and age, childhood, parenthood and adulthood.

Step-by-Step Recovery

It was at that time also that I began to wish with great intensity to get out of the hospital. Moving to the Rehabilitation Ward was a positive step for me, and my memories shift in sharper focus at this time. Getting out of bed and into a wheelchair, moving around the ward, socializing with other patients, and eating my meals in the communal dining room, all helped me to get back into the world of reality. Staff members became individuals, instead of interchangeable; but there was still a degree of fuzziness about my perceptions of people and things at that time. Returning for further surgery months later, when I had regained a much greater degree of functioning, I was astonished at how worn the ward was, housed as it was in the oldest wing of the building. These details had completely escaped my attention before.

It was then, also, that I started to use my adult qualities of judgment for the first time since my accident. Wanting desperately to get out of the hospital, I made a conscious decision that I would play the hospital game in whatever way was necessary to get out. I made sure, for example, that before my doctor's visits I carefully noted the date, day and time, so I could answer his questions. I ate all my meals, I spent hours exercising and practicing with my crutches, I worked hard at physiotherapy and I refused sleeping pills and pain-killers at night; so that there was no danger of sleeping too soundly and wetting the bed.

All of this paid off, for after having spent only two months in the hospital, instead of the eighteen months that had been anticipated, I was allowed to go home. I have to confess that until I saw the inimitable silhouette of the Okanogan Lake Bridge at Kelowna etched on the horizon, I secretly cherished the last of my delusions (that I was still in Kamloops).

The car ride is sharply delineated in my memory. I had great difficulty in visually tracking sights as they whirled past the windows. I felt dazed and stunned by the kaleidoscope of sights and sounds. It felt strange to drive along the streets, unable to remember what came around the corner, yet knowing as soon as I saw it that it was familiar. I have never felt so intensely what it was like to be poised on the knife-edge between known and unknown, with the strangeness turning into familiarity, as the road unreeled before my eyes.

The most intense moment came when we drove into our yard. I had wanted ardently to get home while in the hospital; but home was just an emotional feeling. I had no idea what it looked like. Suddenly there it was, in all its loved reality, with a homemade sign my son had made: 'Welcome Home Dad' flapping from the porch. As I hobbled in, a huge chunk of memories fell into place intact: But these were not just memories of the physical layout of the house, where the things were, and so forth... but also the feelings and emotions that went with them. When I saw the sign, for example, I knew that my son had made it, that 'Dad' was me and I was an adult and a father.

For the next eight months, I recuperated at home before returning back to work. Looking back, I see that I had three problems to deal with. First of all, there was the physical rehabilitation: learning to cope with the casts and crutches and these were eventually discarded, learning to cope with the permanent disabilities that remain. Secondly, there was the task of assessing the brain damage, and **learning to live with and work around the deficits.** Thirdly, there was the process of emotional or psychological healing; building up sufficient confidence in myself to be able to discard the role of the 'handicapped person' and resume the full load of responsibility at work and at home. I had to keep working on all three of these areas at the same time, for lack of progress in one area slowed down progress in the others and vice versa. For example, an arrangement of stout knotted ropes enabled me to pull myself out of bed and the purchase of an electric coffee maker permitted me to get up at my preferred early rising hour and make my own morning coffee, rather than lying helplessly in bed waiting for my wife to wake up and haul me to my feet. This gave me a great psychological lift and spurred me on to other steps of independence. Learning to maneuver safely on crutches led to being able to go shopping, to church, to friends homes, all of which **provided mental stimulation and promoted a return to normalcy.**

Learning to live with the brain damage was, for me, a major area of challenge, and still is. The diagnosis, after extensive testing, was damage to the temporal lobe of

the brain, several cranial nerves and lesser damage to the right parietal area.
Implications

The results of this damage were: lack of taste and smell, impaired short-term auditory and visual memory, lessened emotional control and a greater tendency toward depression. It has been found that damage to the right temporal area of the brain often leaves the sufferer blissfully unaware that there is any deficit, even when it is quite obvious to those around him. Damage to the left temporal area, however, often allows the individual to be keenly aware of his deficits. It was thought that this is why this type of damage predisposes the sufferer to depressions. In my case, **I initially denied that I had any deficits at all**, and it was only after the process of physical and psychological healing was well under way, that I could accept that I had damage in some areas and begin to cope with it. For example, for weeks I denied that I had any loss of taste or smell, yet these senses were, in fact, totally absent for over a year and have only partially returned even two years later.

My short-term visual and auditory memory was severely impaired for a long time. Here again, I initially denied this and it was quite frustrating for my family to tell me things, which I would forget immediately, later on insisting vehemently that I had not been told anything in the first place. Again, I would meet a person for the first time and, seeing them an hour later, fail to recognize them. Or I would read a simple paragraph in the newspaper and by the time I got to the last sentence, have no recollection what the first one was.

Having been a highly self-controlled person all my life, I found myself with a hair-trigger temper and labile emotions. It is theorized that this state is due to CNS irritation or else that some part of the brain, which is responsible for braking the mental motor, is dysfunctional after brain damage has occurred.

A corollary of this deficit is the **perseverance** frequently displayed in brain damaged people, and which I recognize in myself. I realize that I have much more of <u>a one track mind</u> than I used to, and my thinking tends to proceed along linear lines. Possibly, this is due to the deficit in the mental braking process, discussed above. **When once embarked on a train of thought, I find it very hard to stop, deal with a side issue and then return quickly to the original theme. Distractions, either external or internal are hard to handle**...and I find myself most comfortable in dealing with clear cut issues, where I can reason in a straightforward fashion.

Coping Needs

In learning to live with my brain damage, I have found through trial and error, that certain things help greatly and others hinder coping. In order to learn and retain information best, I try to eliminate as many distractions as possible and concentrate all my mental energy to the task at hand. A structured routine, well organized and a serene atmosphere at home and as far as possible at work, is vital to me. In the past, I enjoyed a rather chaotic lifestyle; but now I find I want a place for everything and everything in its place. When remembering is difficult, order and habit make a minutia of daily living much easier.

Coping is also easier in the milieu that is free of emotional tension, competitiveness, anxiety and pressure. I see all of these as distractions, that lessen my ability to learn, just as surely as noise, chaos and change in the physical setting. I find it hard to absorb and retain new information in a meeting with people who are new to me and where there is a constant interchange of ideas and

personalities. Yet in a one-to-one situation with a familiar client, or working in my office with colleagues whom I know and trust, in an orderly and systematic fashion, I can retain far more and function far more effectively. In other words, <u>simplification of the</u> external <u>situation</u>, both physical and emotional, assists me to master new information. The more complexity around me, the less I am able to cope.

I also find that physical fatigue cuts down my concentration and so I now try to tackle new tasks in the morning, when I am physically fresh. I resort to extensive note taking on professional matters, as well as carefully recording all my appointments, financial details and so forth at home. In mastering new information, I go over the subject matter many times, using all possible sensory input channels; reading it, writing it down, repeating it aloud and having someone re-read it to me. These ways of modifying the external environment will, I am convinced, assist and brain damaged person to learn better. From a purely internal point of view, however, I feel that other psychological factors are extremely important.

Understanding the Brain Damaged Person

First of all, any brain damaged person is going to feel some degree of anger, denial and depression as his deficits become apparent. These have to be dealt with if the individual is to succeed in using his fullest potential and in coping with the real world. For example, as I have mentioned, for many weeks I denied that I had lost my sense of taste and smell. I never mentioned the loss to anyone while I was in the hospital...and it was only on the safe ground of home that I took the first steps towards admission of this deficit. This was to complain to my wife that food tasted funny. I accused her of adding something strange to it, and then theorized that she had bought food that wasn't fresh or that had gone bad. Finally, when I was able to accompany her to the store, buy the food myself and be assured of its quality, and do the actual cooking myself, I had to admit that the fault was not in the food itself, but in my own senses. The same process had to be gone through in other areas of deficiency, mental and physical – as I denied the deficits, came up against the hard edge of reality and finally accepted them. Anger and depression inevitably accompany the final admission of such deficits, sometimes separately, sometimes together. I remember periods of intense depression, during which I would retreat to the bedroom for hours on end, covering up my true feelings by saying that the **noise of the children** was too much for me. I was also subject to fits of rage and had a hair-trigger temper, that could be ignited by the smallest incident. This all became so difficult for my family (themselves under great stress), that my wife insisted that we see the psychiatrist who had worked with me while I was in the hospital.

Almost immediately after the interview began, he recognized and pointed out my extreme depression. I broke down and began to weep and it was then that I was able to recognize my feelings for what they actually were. Talking with this understanding doctor, who was familiar with the medical and neurological background of my situation, was of great help in working through my depression. Medication was of help as well; but the important part was seeking help, being able to understand my feelings, and being able to talk about them and express them, in tears if appropriate.

My intense anger was dealt with in the same way. I talked about it with my doctor and my family... and we discussed what situations were most likely to trigger off an explosion, and how to avoid these situations or diffuse them. Medications eased the process, and gradually the anger dissipated.

I have had to recognize, however, that a problem still remains in this area. I cannot cope with anger as well as I was able to before my accident. Rage, related to my losses, does not just lie under the surface waiting to explode as it did earlier in my recovery. Yet, like any other person living in the real world, situations arise which make me justifiably angry, and I am still, today slow to anger. The difference is that now, once I become angry, I find it impossible to put the brakes on and I attribute this directly to my brain damage. It is extremely frightening to me to find myself in this state, and I still have not worked out a truly satisfactory solution; except insofar as I try to avoid anger-provoking situations, or try to deal with them before they become too provoking.

Regaining Independence

In the final analysis, though, the problem was greatly alleviated by my taking on gradually increasing responsibilities, first at home, then at work. Each step gave me a sense of accomplishment and self-confidence. It is salutary to accept one's losses, but there comes a time when one must reaffirm what remains and even begin to explore previously untapped potentials.

In this vein, I have mentioned that being able to get out of bed unassisted and make the morning coffee was a great step for me in the direction of full recovery. Next, I took over the planning and organization of the family's meals, shopping lists, and some <u>limitedcooking</u>. As time went on and I grew stronger, I took over all of the housework, <u>cooking</u>, cleaning, laundry and so forth. I enjoyed doing these things, but at first they were quite an ordeal for the family. A shopping trip that would have taken my wife and hour would occupy an entire morning, with me making laborious lists, checking and rechecking. Let alone the problem of getting me in and out of the car, maneuvering up and down the aisles with crutches, casts and shopping cart to be taken into account.

Yet, looking back, I realize how vital it was for me to feel that I was no longer totally dependent, that I had <u>certain responsibilities and tasks within the home that were mine alone</u>, and that I was to some degree at least justifying my existence.

My family was most supportive, but I remember having to push hard at times against their tendency to overprotect me and treat me as a fragile invalid. In fact, at times

I lost confidence in myself, because they
didn't think I could do something. This is a
sensitive area and one that probably
presents the greatest difficulty for
the families of brain damaged people.
Most families have reserves of compassion
and protectiveness that they can draw on in
dealing with a hurt member. Supporting the
injured one is not hard; it is the letting go
that is difficult. It takes a great deal of
sensitivity and courage for family members
to change roles at the appropriate time and
let the handicapped person go it alone. At
times, it may take the intervention of an
outsider (doctor, friend, colleague), who is
not so emotionally involved to nudge the
family into their new role and allow the
handicapped person to take the next steps on
the road to recovery.
In my case, this happened when I had to
make a decision to resign from my job. I had
no confidence in my abilities to handle the
work again and my wife accepted this. I felt
that it was only fair to any clients and
colleagues that I resign and allow my job to
be filled; so with much sadness I sent in my
letter of resignation.

My director, backed by the rest of the staff,
did something that took courage and
perception. She refused to accept
my **resignation** and after a long emotional

session, somehow gave me the confidence and courage to return to work on a part-time basis. Her confidence was not misplaced; I found that I could handle the work, and thanks to her, retained my job.

I would say that **it is imperative that brain damaged people (especially youngsters who have no previous achievements to fall back upon) be provided with <u>challenges and responsibilities</u>**. What is the point of struggling to learn, to absorb, and to achieve on an intellectual level, when one is not allowed to <u>exercise</u> one's new powers in the real world? Such a person is literally, all dressed up with no place to go.

No matter how hard it is for family members, teachers and others to let the brain damaged person do it on his own, and no matter how much easier, it would be to take pity on them and do it yourself, and **no matter how long it takes, or how messy the job when done, the brain damaged person must keep moving towards the fullest development of his or her potential**. In my own case, without that gradual build-up of confidence in small matters, starting with making that first cup of coffee on my own, I would never have been able to take the final step of going back into full time employment.

Conclusion

In brief then, **I have found that internal and external factors must mesh smoothly in order for the brain damaged person to reach their fullest potential and cope with his/her disabilities. An accurate diagnosis of the deficits must be made and must be understood and accepted by the individual and by those closely involved with their rehabilitation. The individual and family must be motivated to pursue the fullest development of his/her potential. Challenges and responsibilities must be provided as he/she progresses, permitting a growing sense of self-worth and involvement in the real world. Environment at home and at school or work must be structured to maximize learning.**

One last word... **No one really knows just how great an individual's potential is. In my case, I was given a slim chance of survival and it was thought that I would be a human vegetable if I did live. Instead, I am living a full and productive life and in fact, can honestly say that I enjoy it more than I ever did before.** People close to me tell me that I am easier to live with and work with, now that I am not the highly self-controlled person that I used to be. My emotions are more openly displayed and more accessible. Partially due to the brain damage that precludes any storing up of emotion, and partially due to the maturational aspects of this whole life threatening experience. <u>I have come through the crises in my life with more respect for myself and more trust in others.</u> <u>My new openness of feeling makes it easier for me to communicate with others and for others to understand me. People know where they stand with me at all times and trust me more.</u>

-

Furthermore, my blood pressure is amazingly low! My one-track mind seems to help me take each day as it comes without excessive worry, as I enjoy the simple things of life in a way I never did before. As well, I seem to be a more effective therapist, since I stick to the basic issues at hand and have <u>more empathy</u> with others than I did previously.

I do not bewail what I have lost, because I am at <u>peace</u> with myself. I have fought a hard battle, given it my best, and won far more that I or anyone else ever thought I would. I ask only that other brain damaged people be given the chance to fight their battles too, and to find out for

**themselves what their unique
potential is.**
Reprinted 1980 with permission of the
author.

Frederick R. Linge, Clinical Psychologist

and shared by craig ("just an information
and inspiration distributer and people-
builder")

(I found this article very helpful many years
ago, when I felt that my entire life felt
shattered in pieces, like Humpty Dumpty's
great wall. In the deep deep valley Dr Linge's
story had so much meaning for us as a family
(as it expressed so much better than I ever
could exactly how I felt on my own journey
from darkness into the light). Thanks for
sharing your insights, Dr Linge)

*Success to others may be apparent in what
you DO; but significance, meaning and
purpose lies, then reveals itself in what you
ARE and BECOME down the 'river of life' –
how and the spirit with which you face, then
overcome the daily obstacles, the frequent
trials and tribulations along the often rocky
path-way of life's magical and mysterious
journey.Light your path brightly."*
- craig

at and
PS: To end off, enjoy these thoughts...

*"We have it within; but we get it all from
without. There is a well-spring of
strength, <u>wisdom</u>, courage and
great <u>imagination</u> within each one of us;
but once we draw on this truth, it gets
watered from without, by a Higher Source
– the Source of Life and Love, which is God,
the very Ground of our Being."*

*"When you can see no light at the end of the
tunnel, light your own candle and let your
light illuminate the world, like the radiance
from a window at midnight."*
That's a metaphor, BTW"

*"The task ahead of you can always be
overcome by the power within you...and the
seemingly difficult path ahead of you is
never as steep with the great spirit that lies
within you."*
*"When the world is filled with love, people's
hearts are overflowing with hope."*
- craig
This article may be freely reproduced
electronically or in print. If through sharing
a little of my experiences, it helps anyone
"out there in the often very difficult, but

always amazing 'journey of life' in any way, then I'm very happy.

2. Two years after a brain injury left him introverted and aggressive, James Cracknell and his wife Bev tell how it nearly tore them apart

Posted on November 16, 2012by craiglock

Two years after a brain injury left him introverted and aggressive, James Cracknell and his wife Bev tell how it nearly tore them apart

By Rebecca Hardy
From http://www.dailymail.co.uk/femail/article-2226360/James-Cracknell-wife-Beverley-tell-brain-injury-nearly-tore-apart.html
PUBLISHED: 17:25 GMT, 4 November 2012 | **UPDATED:** 17:25 GMT, 4 November 2012

- Comments (0)
- Share

Olympic rower James Cracknell and his wife Beverley have talked about little else in the past two years besides whether they can hold their marriage together. They're still not sure.

The other weekend they celebrated their tenth wedding anniversary with a night away at a hotel in Richmond, south-west London.

It was one of the few grown-up times they've had together without their three children – Croyde, nine, Kiki, three, and 18-month-old Trixie – since James suffered a brain injury after being whacked on the back of the head by the wing mirror of a petrol tanker while cycling in Arizona.

James and Beverley are still unsure of whether they can hold their marriage down

'It was awkward,' says James, 40. 'It was really nice to get away, but there was also that realisation that we hadn't had time alone together for so long so it felt very unusual. It was a lesson we should do it more often. If I don't make an effort, the reality is I may not have my family in the future.

'That would be the worst outcome – if we don't stay together.' And, for a man who struggles to show emotion since his brain injury, James looks indescribably sad.

It was in July 2010 that the double Olympic rowing gold medallist was hit by a truck while attempting to travel from Los Angeles to New York in 16 days – running, cycling, rowing and swimming.

More...

- <u>Laura Carmichael- Downton Abbey's Lady Edith- on her humble beginnings, hanging out with her screen sisters, and how Julian Fellowes discovered a country pile hidden in her past</u>
- <u>Former racing driver, Sir Stirling Moss, 82, relives the horrific crash 50 years ago that put an end to his career</u>
- <u>Martin Shaw's no fan of reality TV, but accepting an offer to mentor an amateur dramatic society for a new show had a profound effect on him</u>

His brain smashed against the front of his skull, damaging the frontal lobe – the part of the brain that governs personality.

When the call came, Beverley, now 38, didn't know whether her husband would be paralysed, brain-damaged or even dead by the time she got to the hospital. Ten days later, she discovered she was pregnant with Trixie, at a time when the doctors were unable to tell her if James would ever be the same again.

Even now, two years later, he is not. Beverley has struggled to recognise the 'gentle, laid-back, surferish' James she married. Instead, she has had to contend with an irritable, occasionally aggressive stranger. It became impossible to leave James and Croyde in the same room together because this once-besotted dad would bully and mock his son.

Beverley didn't know whether her husband would be paralysed, brain-damaged or even dead by the time she got to the hospital

'That was when I was almost going to ring his parents and say, "You're going to have to take him. I can't have him near the children." That was my red flag,' Beverley says.

'I don't know why I didn't. I just felt sorry for him as well. It wasn't his fault. But in that first year I wasn't sure I could do this for the rest of my life. No woman would be. No matter how much you love them, that person is effectively dead.

'I remember being in a supermarket and Sade's By Your Side was playing. It was the song we walked down the aisle to. I stood in the cereal aisle and had a bit of a weep to myself. It was just so heartbreaking, thinking, "This is rubbish. I'm buying food for the house. I've got to go to pick the children up from school. James is at home, but he can't help me because he can't drive."

'It sounds silly, but it's the trivial practicalities that make you feel really alone. He couldn't support me. He was the one person I wanted to talk to about how messed up the situation was, but he was the one person I couldn't discuss it with.'

Beverley, a former competitive swimmer and television presenter, is a bright, feisty, no-nonsense Northerner. She's a stayer, not a bolter, but those first 18 months were enough to test the patience of a saint. James's temper was explosive, and when Beverley was barely four months pregnant he lost it completely and tried to throttle her.

She details these horrifying times with huge poignancy in the book they've written together, Touching Distance. So much so that when James read his wife's words shortly before the book went to the printers, he added to the dedication, 'For Croyde, Kiki, Trixie; all of our amazing family... and every person whose life is touched by brain injury. (And Bev, it's only from reading your words that I truly understand what you've been through. I adore you.)'

For such is the nature of James's injury he cannot remember much of what happened in the first year or so after his accident. 'I'm generally not someone who shows emotion,'

he says, 'but I couldn't read more than a few
pages without crying.

'The worst thing was reading how scared Bev
was.' As he says this he looks beseechingly at
his wife, who reaches out to touch his hand.
'Even if I have been angry with our son, I've
never smacked him and I've never hit Bev.
To think I'd put someone I loved in that
position...' He shakes his head.

While Beverley feels extremely sorry for her
husband, she began to doubt whether she
could continue to be with him

The divorce rate among couples dealing with
brain injury is 75 per cent and James is
desperate not to be another statistic. 'I cope
better now but I can remember situations
where I've felt frustrated,' he says. 'I couldn't
understand why I wasn't being understood.
Through my eyes everything looked vaguely
as it had done before the accident. It was
other people who were treating me
differently.'

The truth is, James's behaviour was bizarre
in the first months. He convinced himself
he'd been commissioned to ghost-write Gary
Lineker's column on the Ryder Cup, telling
Beverley, 'His girlfriend told me because she

slept in my room last night.' But he's come on in leaps and bounds.

Today, his eyes sparkle and his wit is quick. Take, for example, when he explains that tests show his ability to recognise faces is towards the special needs end of the scale, whereas his numerical recall is up there with members of Mensa, Nasa and MI6. Ever fancied being a spy James?

'Well, maybe James Bond,' he says. 'But I wouldn't be able to tell the baddies from the goodies.' We both laugh, then he adds, 'I've had to recognise I've changed.'

The divorce rate among couples dealing with brain injury is 75 per cent and James is desperate not to be another statistic

So has Beverley. 'When we were first home I thought, "He's never going to bear any resemblance to the person I married." That was a bleak time. I thought, "I'm going to have to start grieving."' I wonder what's left to love when the man she knew has gone.

'I have a great respect for him for doing everything he's doing [meetings for future documentaries, commentating during the Olympics]. He could have so easily laid on

the sofa for two years and felt sorry for
himself.

'And I do still fancy him, he's still in great
physical shape and he makes me laugh every
day,' she grins. 'I didn't fancy him for a
while because brain injury complicates how
you see that person. But there were much
bigger issues to worry about than the
physical side of our relationship.

'That was probably when our relationship
was less like that of husband and wife, when
he was home for the first year to 18 months
and was in a bleak place. He just wasn't
funny any more because he didn't find life
funny. Weeks went by when he didn't seem
to smile, let alone laugh. In that situation
you think, "How am I going to ever be back
on an even keel?"'

Working together on their book has been a
huge help. 'I've got to spend more time with
him and I'm able to see his personality again.
I think he'll always be different, but I'm
beginning to see 'different' might not
necessarily be bad.

'There's not a day goes by when we don't
wish this hadn't happened, but we've got to
try and see it in a positive way. If nothing
else I think about the families who are living

with brain injuries who can read this book.
All marriages can be difficult, but you stick
with it because that's what you do – until
you get to a point where you really can't do
that any more.'

But after spending several hours with this
gutsy couple, I wouldn't mind betting that
won't be any time soon.

***Touching Distance by James
Cracknell and Beverley Turner,
published by Century in hardback
and ebook, £18.99.***
Read
more: http://www.dailymail.co.uk/femail/ar
ticle-2226360/James-Cracknell-wife-
Beverley-tell-brain-injury-nearly-tore-
apart.html#ixzz2CP3RdRRt
Follow us: @MailOnline on
Twitter | DailyMail on Facebook
Also
see http://news.bbc.co.uk/2/hi/programme
s/hardtalk/9769816.stm
James Cracknell: Brain injury
changed my personality

The double gold medal winning Olympic
rower, James Cracknell tells Stephen Sackur
how an accident which left him with a brain
injury has changed his life and put his family
relationships under strain.

In July 2010, Mr Cracknell was hit from behind by a petrol tanker whilst cycling during an attempt to cycle, row, run and swim from Los Angeles to New York within 16 days.

He told the BBC's Hardtalk programme about how his injury has affected his relationship with his son and his wife.

If you have had a similar experience with Traumatic Brain Injury (TBI) a research team for a BBC documentary currently in development would be interested in hearing from you. Please email: kathleen.mullin@bbc.co.uk You can watch the full interview on BBC World News on Thursday 15 November at 04:30, 09:30, 15:30 and 21:30 GMT and the BBC News Channel at 0030 and 0430 GMT on Friday 16 November 2012 and 0030 on Saturday 17 November 2012
Watch **recent episodes** online (UK only) or subscribe to our podcast. Find out who is coming up on the programme by following us on **Twitter** .

from http://www.jamescracknell.com and http://thedriverthenurseandthewriter.wordpress.com/

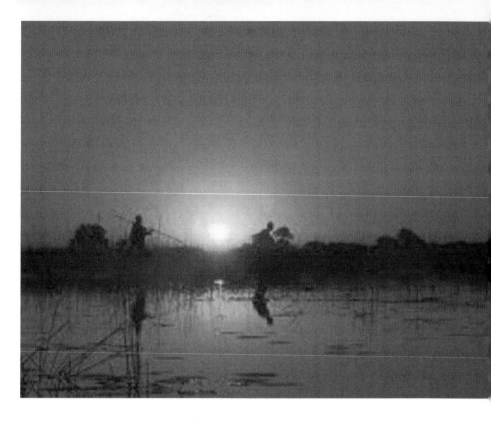

"Do not what you can't do stop you from doing what you CAN do …best!"

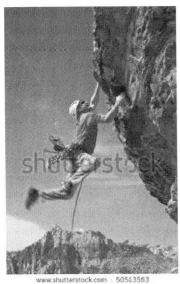

"Do not what you can't do stop you from doing what you CAN do ...best!"
- me (as inspired by the words of John Wooten)

from https://craigsquotes.wordpress.com/
PS

This "non-techno" is just learning about videos
see http://raceinthezone.wordpress.com/2014/08/29/the-greatest-race-living-by-with-faith-hope-and-love-is-the-highest-podium-any-person-can-reach-gods-podium-that-anyone-stand-on-2/
enjoy
"Together, one mind, one life at a time, let's see how many people we can impact, empower, uplift and

encourage to reach their fullest potentials."

The various books* that Craig "felt inspired to write" are available athttp://www.amazon.com/s/ref=la_B005G GMAW4_sr?rh=i%3Abooks&field-author=Craig+Lock http://www.amazon.com/-/e/B005GGMAW4 http://www.creativekis.com/amazon.htmland http://goo.gl/vTpjk http://www.amazon.com/dp/B007E2WXW0

All proceeds go to needy and underprivileged children -

MINE!

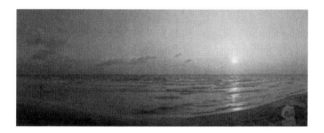

"Every adversity, every failure, every heartache carries with it the seed of an equal or greater benefit."

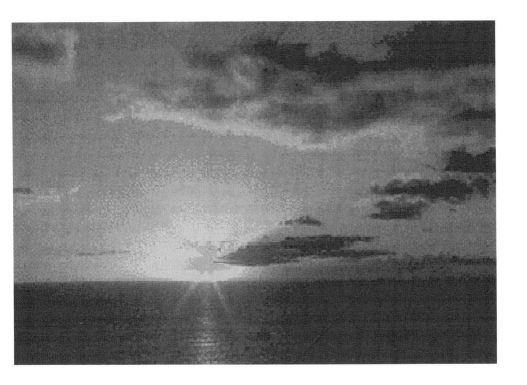

"Every adversity, every failure, every heartache carries with it the seed* of an equal or greater benefit."
– Napoleon Hill (in his great book '**Think** and Grow Rich')
* this should perhaps read "rather the POTENTIAL seed" in cases of head (brain) damage

"Just because a brain has been damaged, does NOT necessarily have to affect the human mind...and so the quality and height of our thoughts!"
"Let's not what we can't do stop us from doing what we CAN do...best!"
"The only limits are the ones we hold in our own minds."

"There are no perceived limits,
just horizons far and wide...endless
and great possibilities"
- craig

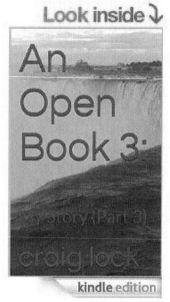

from http://www.amazon.com/An-Open-Book-little-Story/dp/1500769347
and following on
from http://craigsbooks.wordpress.com/2014/08/07/an-open-book-books-1-and-2-3/
PPS

You may also like my new video
at https://livingwithheadinjury.wordpress.com/
and

see http://raceinthezone.wordpress.com/2014/08/29/the-greatest-race-living-by-with-faith-hope-and-love-is-the-highest-podium-

THE FINAL WORD

*: Do not what you can't do – stop
what you CAN do… best!*

*"I do not bewail what I have lost, because I
am at peace with myself. I have fought a
hard battle, given it my best, and won far
more that I or anyone else ever thought I
would. I ask only that other brain damaged
people be given the chance to fight their
battles too, and to find out for themselves
what their unique potential is."*
– Frederick Linge

."
- *- c*

*Do not what you can't do – stop what
you CAN do… best!*

From An Open Book (paperback published by
Createspace)

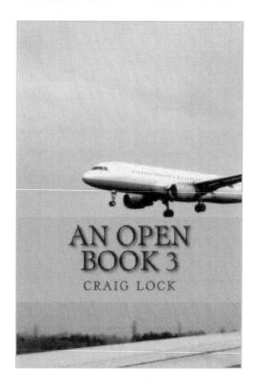

http://www.amazon.com/Open-Book-little-Story-Book3/dp/1500769347/

and

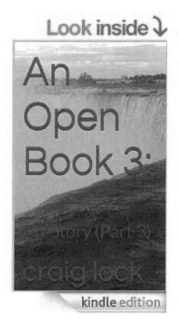

at http://www.amazon.com/An-Open-Book-Story-Part-ebook/dp/B00MD4U9QQ

*"The past is history, the future is a mystery,
and this moment is
the gift, that is why this moment is called the
present."*

- anon

from
http://www.selfgrowth.com/articles/how_mak
e_good_life_decisions_updated.html

WHAT IS SUCCESS?

*To laugh often and much;
To win the respect of intelligent people and the
affection of children;
To earn the appreciation of honest critics and
endure the betrayal of false friends;
To appreciate beauty, to find the best in others;
To leave the world a bit better, whether by a
healthy child, a garden patch or a redeemed
social condition;
To know even one life has breathed easier
because you have lived.
This is to have succeeded.*
-    Ralph Waldo Emerson (1803 - 1882)

**"Together, one mind, one life (one small
step at a time), let's see how many people
(and lives) we can encourage, impact,
empower, enrich, uplift and perhaps even
inspire to reach their fullest
potentials...and strive for and perhaps**

one sunny day even achieve their wildest
dreams."

THE END

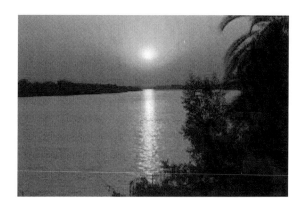

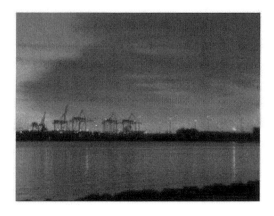

Printed in Poland
by Amazon Fulfillment
Poland Sp. z o.o., Wrocław

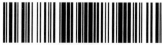

49690463R00049